25 Low Calories Foods And Their Recipes

The best foods

For losing weight and the easiest recipes

you should try

Table of contents

Iced Coffee

10. GRAPEFRUIT

Grapefruit, Walnut, and Feta Salad
Avocado Cucumber Grapefruit Salad
Grapefruit Spinach Salad Recipe

11. MUSHROOMS

Stuffed Masala Mushrooms
Mushroom Pasta
Cream of Mushroom & Barley Soup

12. TOMATOES

Tomato Salad with Edamame
Tropical Tomato Salsa
Roasted Tomato Basil Pesto Pasta

13. ZUCCHINI

Sautéed Zucchini
Ratatouille
Coconut Chickpea Curry

14. SPINACH

Fresh Spinach Dip
Strawberry Spinach Salad
Spinach Soup

15. LEMONS AND LIMES

Lime soda
Healthy Baked Lemon Chicken
Lemon Bars

16. KALE

Kale With Roasted Peppers and Olives
Vegetable Barley Soup
Kale Smoothie

17. GARLIC

Garlic & Herb Yogurt Dip
Garlic Bread
Mussels with Garlic

18. PEPPERS

Baked Eggs in Stuffed Peppers with Butternut Squash Hash
Spicy Red Pepper Sauce
Spicy Sausage And Pepper Pasta

19. ONIONS

French onion soup
Tomato, red onion and balsamic salsa
Glazed onions

20. PUMPKIN

Coconut Curry Pumpkin Soup
Pumpkin Biscuits
Pumpkin-Apple Butter

21. RADISHES

Indian Spiced Radishes & Pumpkin
Roasted Radishes

22. FENNEL

Roasted Squash, Onion And Fennel Toss
Apple Fennel Celery Salad
Fennel & White Bean Pasta

23. CELERY

Celery Salad
Celery Stir Fry
Spicy Shrimp, Celery, and Cashew Stir-fry

24. BERRIES

Triple Berry Banana Yogurt Smoothie
Greek Yogurt Berry Medley Smoothie

25. CARROTS

Carrot Cake
Honey Glazed Carrots
Roasted Carrots

Asparagus

Calories: 27 per cup

Asparagus is traditionally known as a detoxifying food, because it contains high levels of an amino acid that acts as a diuretic, flushing excess fluid out of your system. It also helps speed the metabolism of alcohol and other toxins.

Asparagus is also a powerhouse of vitamins and minerals, including vitamins A, C, E, and K, B6, folate, iron, copper, and even protein. We love the tender shoots in their most natural form, raw and tossed into salads, or steamed.

Asparagus Salad With Sweet Balsamic Vinegar

Ingredients

1/3 cup balsamic vinegar
3 tablespoons olive oil
1 tablespoon Dijon mustard
1 tablespoon chopped fresh marjoram or 1 teaspoon dried
1 teaspoon minced garlic
2 pounds asparagus, tough ends trimmed, cut on diagonal into 2-inch pieces
1 small red bell pepper, diced
1/3 cup chopped pecans, toasted

Preparation

Boil vinegar in heavy small saucepan over medium heat until reduced by half, about 3 minutes. Pour vinegar into large bowl. Whisk in oil, mustard, marjoram and garlic. Season dressing to taste with salt and pepper.
Cook asparagus in large pot of boiling salted water until crisp-tender, about 4 minutes. Drain; rinse with cold water and drain again. Add asparagus and bell pepper to dressing; toss to blend well. Sprinkle with pecans and serve.

Asparagus And Mixed Greens Salad

Ingredients

2 teaspoons olive oil
1 cup pecan pieces
1 bunch asparagus (1 lb/450 g), trimmed
1 pinch salt
1 pinch pepper
4 cups torn frisée lettuce
4 cups baby arugula leaves
4 cups trimmed watercress
1 head boston lettuce torn
Lemon Fennel Vinaigrette:
1/4 cup olive oil
3 tablespoons minced shallots
3 tablespoons lemon juice
2 teaspoons liquid honey
2 teaspoons Dijon mustard
1 1/2 teaspoon crushed fennel seeds
1/2 teaspoon salt
1/2 teaspoon pepper

Preparation

On baking sheet, bake pecans in 350°F (180°C) oven until lightly toasted, about 8 minutes. Let cool. (Make-ahead: Store in airtight container for up to 5 days.)

Lemon Fennel Vinaigrette: Meanwhile, in small bowl, whisk together oil, shallot, lemon juice, honey, mustard, fennel seeds, salt and pepper. Set aside. (Make-ahead: Refrigerate in airtight container for up to 3 days.)

Toss asparagus with oil, salt and pepper. Bake on rimmed baking sheet in 350°F (180°C) oven until tender-crisp, 6 to 8 minutes. Let cool; cover and refrigerate. (Make-ahead: Refrigerate in airtight container for up to 24 hours.)

Arrange asparagus on salad plates. In large bowl, toss together pecans, frisée, arugula, watercress, Boston lettuce and vinaigrette. Divide over asparagus. Serve immediately.

Cherry Tomato and Asparagus Salad

Ingredients

1 pound asparagus, trimmed and halved
6 cups halved cherry, grape, and pear tomatoes in varied colors
1/2 cup crumbled gorgonzola cheese
1 ripe avocado, cut into cubes
1 cup sliced basil leaves
1/4 cup extra-virgin olive oil
2 teaspoons lemon juice
2 teaspoons Dijon mustard
1/2 teaspoon kosher salt
1/2 teaspoon pepper

Preparation

1. Boil asparagus in a large pot of salted water for 2 minutes. Drain and rinse with cold water.

2. Mix asparagus with remaining ingredients in a large bowl, stirring well to coat evenly with dressing.

Broccoli

Calories: 31 per cup

Broccoli is amazingly low in calories, but it always makes our list of the top superfoods for a reason. Not only is it packed with fiber, vitamins, and minerals, it contains powerful antioxidants that may improve your odds of breast cancer survival and reduce the risk of colon cancer.

The chemical in broccoli responsible for the protective effect is called sulforaphane, and yes, it gives broccoli its slightly bitter flavor.

Broccoli Salad

Ingredients

1/2 cup Miracle Whip Original Spread
1/2 cup sugar
2 Tbsp. Heinz Distilled White Vinegar
12 cups broccoli florets
1 small red onion, finely chopped
1/2 cup raisins
1/4 cup sunflower kernels
5 slices bacon, cooked, crumbled

Preparation

Mix Miracle Whip, sugar and vinegar.
Combine broccoli, onions, raisins and sunflower kernels in large bowl. Add Miracle Whip mixture; toss to coat.
Refrigerate several hours. Sprinkle with bacon before serving.

Sunflower Seeds & Cranberries Broccoli Salad

Ingredients

2-3 broccoli crowns, just the florets, finely chopped (5-6 cups)
10 bacon slices, crisp-cooked and crumbled
1/3c red onion, diced
1/3c sunflower seeds
1/3c dried cranberries, chopped (golden raisins are equally good)
1/2c mayonnaise
2T apple cider vinegar
2t sugar
salt and pepper

Preparation

To a salad bowl, add broccoli, bacon, onion, seeds, and cranberries. In a small bowl, mix mayo, vinegar, and sugar. Pour dressing mixture over salad and toss to coat. Season with salt and pepper to taste. Cover and refrigerate until ready to serve (at least one hour).

Classic Broccoli Cheddar Soup

Ingredients

1 bunch broccoli
1 medium onion, chopped
2 small baking potatoes, peeled and diced
1 clove garlic, minced
2 cups (500 mL) reduced-sodium chicken or vegetable broth
1 tsp (2 mL) grated orange rind
1/2 tsp (2 mL) dried thyme
1/4 tsp (1 mL) pepper
pinch hot pepper flakes
2 cups (500 mL) milk
1/2 tsp (2 mL) salt
1 cup (250 mL) shredded Cheddar

Preparation

Peel and chop broccoli stems and coarsely chop florets, keeping stems and florets separate (you should have about 6 cups/1.5 L total).

In a pot, combine broccoli stems, onion, potatoes, garlic, broth, orange rind, thyme, pepper and hot pepper flakes; bring to boil. Reduce heat, cover and simmer for 10 min. Add florets; simmer, covered, for 5 min or until vegetables are softened.

Transfer to a blender or food processor, in batches, or use an immersion blender in the pot and purée soup, adding milk, until smooth. Return to pot, if necessary. Heat over medium heat, stirring, until steaming, but do not let boil. Stir in more milk if soup is too thick. Season with up to 1/2 tsp (2 mL) salt. Ladle into bowls; sprinkle with cheese.

Broth

Calories: 10 per cup

Clear beef, chicken, miso, seafood, or vegetable broth is a dieter's secret weapon, nourishing and filling your body for almost zero calories, especially if you toss in leafy greens and lean meat. Broth is the ultimate "high volume food," meaning you can eat large amounts for very few calories and still feel full. It all comes down to calories per bite, or in this case, slurp.

By choosing foods that have fewer calories per bite, your portion size grows, but your overall calorie count decreases, so you end up with a satisfying amount of food.

Cream Of Wild Mushroom Soup

Ingredients

Cream of Mushroom Soup
1 ½ lb   (675 g) white mushrooms, quartered
1 large onion, chopped
3 tbsp   (42 g) butter
5 cups   (1.25 litres) chicken broth
1 small potato, peeled and cubed
6 tbsp (14 g) dried porcini mushrooms, coarsely chopped
Salt and pepper

Topping
3 porcini mushrooms, fresh or frozen and thawed, sliced
2 tbsp (28 g) butter
4 oz (115 g) mixed wild mushrooms of your choice
2 tbsp small flat-leaf parsley leaves
1 tbsp fresh chives, chopped

Preparation

Cream of Mushroom Soup

In a pot over medium heat, brown the mushrooms and onion in the butter. Continue cooking until the mushrooms are caramelized and the juices have completely evaporated. Add the broth, potatoes and dried mushrooms. Bring to a boil.
Cover and simmer about 20 minutes or until the potatoes are tender.
In a blender, purée the soup until smooth. Return to the saucepan. Season with salt and pepper. Keep warm.

Topping

In a large non-stick skillet over medium heat, brown the porcini mushrooms in the butter. Add the remaining mushrooms and cook until they have softened. Season with salt and pepper.
Pour the mushroom soup into bowls. Top with the sautéed mushrooms. Garnish with the fresh herbs.

Vegetable And Fava Bean Soup

Ingredients

1 onion, chopped
2 tbsp (30 ml) olive oil
2 carrots, peeled and cut into small pieces
2 stalks celery, cut into small pieces
1/2 rutabaga, peeled and cut into small pieces
1 can (796 ml/28 oz) plum tomatoes, diced
5 cups (1.25 litres) chicken broth
1 cup (135 g) frozen fava beans, shelled and peeled
Salt and pepper

Preparation

In a saucepan over medium heat, soften the onion in the oil. Add the carrots, celery and rutabaga. Continue cooking for 5 minutes. Add the tomatoes and broth and bring to a boil.

Cover and simmer over low heat for about 40 minutes or until the vegetables are tender. Season with salt and pepper. Add the beans and cook for 2 to 5 minutes or until tender.

Bacon and Egg Drop Soup

Ingredients

4 cups chicken broth
2 cloves garlic, minced
2 stalks scallions, minced
1 1/2 tsp grated fresh ginger
1/4 tsp ground nutmeg
6 strips bacon, chopped into 1-inch pieces
soy sauce, to taste
red chili flakes, to taste
1 tsp black pepper
2 tsp cornstarch
3 eggs

Preparation

combine the first 8 ingredients plus 1/2 teaspoon of black pepper in a large saucepan over medium high heat. bring to a boil and then reduce to a simmer. cover and simmer for 20 minutes.

in a small bowl, stir together the cornstarch with 2 tablespoons of broth. set aside.

in another bowl, beat eggs with remaining 1/2 teaspoon of black pepper. slowly drizzle into the soup, stirring gently. and then slowly stir in the cornstarch mixture.

taste to adjust seasonings, and enjoy!

Brussel sprouts

Calories: 38 per cup

Brussels sprouts are super-low in calories but loaded with cancer-preventing phytonutrients and fiber. These veggies, sometimes called little cabbages, get a bad rap, but they taste great with a sweet or tangy sauce.

Roasted Brussels Sprouts with Bacon, Pecans & Maple Syrup

Ingredients

1/2 cup pecans
6 slices bacon
2 pounds brussels sprouts, halved (stem and ragged outer leaves removed)
3 tablespoons extra virgin olive oil
1 teaspoon kosher salt
1/2 teaspoon freshly ground black pepper
2-1/2 tablespoons balsamic vinegar
1 tablespoon maple syrup

Preparation

Preheat oven to 350 degrees.

Bake pecans until lightly toasted and fragrant, about 5 minutes. Keep a close eye on them, as they can burn fast. Chop the pecans coarsely. Set aside.

Turn the oven heat up to 400 degrees. Roast bacon for 12-20 minutes, rotating the pan from front to back midway through, until the bacon is crisp. Transfer bacon to a plate lined with paper towels; pour rendered bacon fat into a small dish. When bacon is cool, finely chop.

Turn the oven heat up to 425 degrees. Toss the brussels sprouts with the rendered bacon fat, olive oil, salt and pepper directly on the baking sheet. Roast, stirring midway through with rubber spatula to promote even browning, until brussels sprouts are tender and caramelized, about 20 minutes. Add balsamic vinegar and maple syrup and toss to coat evenly. Taste and adjust seasoning, then transfer to a serving dish. Right before serving, top with chopped pecans and bacon. Serve hot or warm.

Pasta With Roasted Cauliflower and Brussels Sprouts

Ingredients

3/4pound rigatoni or some other short pasta
1/2 medium head cauliflower (about 1 pound), cut into florets
8ounces Brussels sprouts, trimmed and halved (quartered if large)
1 medium red onion, cut into 1/2-inch wedges
2 sprigs fresh thyme
4tablespoons olive oil
kosher salt and black pepper
2ounces grated pecorino (about 1/2 cup), plus more for serving

Preparation

Heat oven to 450° F. Cook the pasta according to the package directions. Reserve 1 cup of the cooking water; drain the pasta and return it to the pot.

Meanwhile, on 2 large rimmed baking sheets, toss the cauliflower, Brussels sprouts, and onion with the thyme, 2 tablespoons of the oil, and ½ teaspoon each salt and pepper. Roast, tossing the vegetables once and rotating the sheets halfway through, until golden brown and tender, 15 to 20 minutes.

Add the vegetables, pecorino, ½ cup of the reserved cooking water, and the remaining 2 tablespoons of oil to the pasta and toss to combine (add more cooking water if the pasta seems dry). Serve sprinkled with additional pecorino.

Herbed Chicken Cutlets With Roasted Winter Vegetables

Ingredients

1pound Brussels sprouts, trimmed and halved
1/2 medium head cauliflower, cut into small florets (about 4 cups)
3tablespoons olive oil
kosher salt and black pepper
8 small chicken cutlets (about 11/2 pounds)
1tablespoon herbes de Provence

Preparation

Heat oven to 425° F. On a large rimmed baking sheet, toss the Brussels sprouts and cauliflower with 2 tablespoons of the oil and ½ teaspoon each salt and pepper. Roast, tossing once, until tender, 20 to 25 minutes.
Meanwhile, heat the remaining tablespoon of oil in a large skillet over medium heat. Season the chicken with the herbes de Provence, ½ teaspoon salt, and ¼ teaspoon pepper. Working in batches, cook until golden brown and cooked through, 2 to 3 minutes per side, adding more oil as necessary. Serve with the vegetables.

Cabbage

Calories: 22 per cup

Crunchy, sweet, and affordable! How can a food that is so humble, with so few calories, be so incredibly good for you? Cabbage packs vitamins, minerals, fibers, and several phytonutrients thought to prevent cancer. Glucosinolate is a metabolic detoxifier and sulphoraphane is a powerful anti-carcinogenic.

Purple cabbage also contains anthocyanins and other natural chemicals that boost cellular repair and block cancer growth.

Sauteed Purple Cabbage

Ingredients

2 tablespoons canola oil
1 small onion, sliced
1/2 Purple cabbage, shredded
2 tbsp soy sauce
1/3 cup white or apple cider vinegar
2 tbsp sugar
Salt and pepper

Preparation

Heat a skillet over medium high heat. Add oil and onion and saute 2 minutes. Add cabbage and turn in pan, sauteing it until it wilts, 3 to 5 minutes. Add soy sauce and vinegar to the pan and turn the cabbage in it. Sprinkle sugar over the cabbage and turn again. Season with salt and pepper and reduce heat a bit. Let cabbage continue to cook 10 minutes or until ready to serve, stirring occasionally.

Purple Cabbage & Pecan Salad

Ingredients

Half head cabbage, shredded or 1 bag coleslaw mix
1 cup pecans (better use sweetened pecans)
3 scallions, chopped including the green part

Dressing
1/2 cup vinegar
1/2 cup sugar
1/4 cup oil
1/4 cup soy sauce

Preparation

Mix the dressing well and pour over the cabbage, pecans, and scallions.
Mix well to coat and serve immediately or else the pecans will start to soften.

Purple Cabbage Poriyal

Ingredients

2 1/2 cups shredded Purple cabbage
2 tbsp Fresh peas
Salt & water as needed
2 tbsp canola oil -
1/2 tsp Mustard seeds
1 Big onion, finely chopped
1 Green chilli, slit

Seasonings
3 tbsp Grated coconut
1/2 tsp Coriander seeds
1/2 tsp cumin seeds
1 tsp chili powder
2 tbsp garlic powder

Preparation

Heat a skillet and add oil, saute the big onions and green chilli. After onions turn transparent, add cabbage and fresh peas. Add salt and saute for few minutes in medium flame. After they shrink, sprinkle some water, stir well. Lower the heat and cover with a lid for 10mins.Take care cabbage should not be burnt.

Add seasonings to the cooked cabbage and stir well for few minutes till u get a nice aroma. Serve with rice.

Lettuce

Calories: 5 per cup

You can literally eat pounds of any variety of lettuce and never gain an ounce. Romaine lettuce alone is a great source of vitamin B, folic acid, and manganese, which helps regulate blood sugar and is essential for proper immune system function.

Choose other dark green or purple varieties such as green or red leaf for the most nutrients, and toss with a zesty homemade vinaigrette.

Red-Leaf Lettuce With Shallot Vinaigrette

Ingredients

1 large shallot, minced
2 teaspoons white-wine vinegar
2 teaspoons Dijon mustard
3 1/2 tablespoons olive oil
coarse salt to taste
1 large head red-leaf lettuce

Preparation

Stir together shallot and vinegar and let stand 10 minutes. Whisk in mustard, oil, kosher salt, and pepper to taste until blended. Tear lettuce into bite-size pieces and toss with shallot vinaigrette.

Green Leaf and Mandarin Salad Recipe

Ingredients

8 cups torn green leaf lettuce
1 can (15 ounces) mandarin oranges, drained
1/2 cup crumbled feta cheese
1/4 cup chopped sweet yellow pepper
1/4 cup chopped sweet red pepper
5 tablespoons olive oil
2 tablespoons honey
4-1/2 teaspoons cider vinegar
2 teaspoons Dijon mustard
1/8 teaspoon salt
2 tablespoons finely chopped red onion
1/3 cup sliced almonds, toasted

Preparation

In a salad bowl, combine the lettuce, oranges, cheese and peppers.
In another bowl, whisk the oil, honey, vinegar, mustard and salt. Stir in onion. Pour over salad and toss to coat. Sprinkle with almonds. Serve immediately.

Red-Leaf Salad with Roasted Sweet Potatoes

Ingredients

2 sweet potatoes, peeled and cut into 1-inch chunks
1 medium red onion, quartered
2 tablespoons olive oil
Coarse salt and ground pepper
1 package (10 ounces) frozen cut green beans, thawed
1/3 cup walnuts
1 cup plain low-fat yogurt
2 tablespoons white-wine vinegar
1 garlic clove, crushed through a garlic press
1 head (10 ounces) red-leaf lettuce, torn into bite-size pieces

Preparation

Preheat oven to 450 degrees. On a large rimmed baking sheet, toss together sweet potatoes, onion, and oil; season with salt and pepper. Roast until sweet potatoes are tender, about 20 minutes.

Add green beans and walnuts to sheet; toss. Roast until green beans are tender, about 5 minutes.

Meanwhile, in a small bowl, whisk together yogurt, vinegar, and garlic; season dressing with salt and pepper. Top lettuce with roasted vegetable mixture; drizzle with dressing.

Beets

Calories: 37 per 1/2 cup

Beets are sweet but have very few calories—so you can have something sweet without the guilt. They also are rich in cancer-fighting antioxidants.

Beyond their rich, earthy deliciousness, beets are also a nutritional powerhouse. Rich in iron, fiber, folate, and potassium, they're an excellent way to boost the nutrition in a salad or pasta dish. They get their gorgeous color from betanin, a potent antioxidant.

Beet Chips

Ingredients

3 medium-large beets, rinsed and scrubbed
Olive or canola oil
Sea Salt + Black Pepper
2-3 sprigs rosemary, roughly chopped

Preparation

Preheat oven to 375 degrees F and place oven rack in the center of the oven.

Thinly slice beets with a mandolin (or a sharp knife), getting them as consistently thin as possible. They should curl a little when cut. This will ensure even baking and crispiness.

Divide between two baking sheets and spray or very lightly drizzle with oil. Add a pinch of salt and the rosemary. Toss to coat, then arrange in a single layer, making sure the slices aren't touching.

Bake for 15-20 minutes or until crispy and slightly brown. Be sure to watch closely past the 15 minute mark as they can burn quickly.

Remove from oven, let cool. Then serve.

Beet, Carrot and Pomegranate Salad

Ingredients

4 beets, cooked and peeled
2 medium carrots, peeled
1/2 cup pomegranate seeds
1½ tablespoons red wine
1½ tablespoons red wine vinegar
1 tablespoon honey
1/4 cup extra virgin olive oil
1/4 cup pistachios, chopped
1 tablespoon chives, chopped
1 tablespoon fresh flat leaf parsley, chopped
Salt and pepper to taste

Preparation

Slice the beets and carrots thinly using a mandoline or hand held slicer. Layer on a plate or platter, alternating beets and carrots, sprinkle with pomegranate seeds and set aside.

Mix the red wine, vinegar and honey in a medium bowl. Slowly drizzle in the olive oil while whisking continuously.

Drizzle the dressing on the vegetables to coat. Add pistachios, chives and parsley. Season with flaked salt and freshly ground black pepper and serve immediately or at room temperature.

Beet and Goat Cheese Hummus

Ingredients

1 large beet
1 can chickpeas
2 lemons
1/4 cup tahini paste
1 tsp salt
4 oz. crumbled goat cheese
1/4 cup olive oil
1 tsp cumin

Preparation

First scrub the beet and chop into large cubes. Bake in aluminum foil or on a baking tray at 400°F until soft enough to pierce with a fork (about 25-30 minutes). Allow the beet to cool. In a food processor combine the beet, the rinsed chickpeas, juice from two lemons, tahini paste, salt and goat cheese. Pulse until well blended. Now while the food processor is running drizzle in the olive oil. Blend until smooth.

Cauliflower

Like other cruciferous veggies, cauliflower is full of cancer-fighting phytonutrients and is a great source of vitamin C and folate. Nibble on raw or lightly steamed florets to maximize cauliflower's nutritional power. Cauliflower is one of the top superfoods, that may improve your odds for breast cancer survival.

Curried Cauliflower & Quinoa Salad

Ingredients

1 cauliflower, cut into bite-size florets
2 tsp mustard
2 tsp cumin
1 tsp paprika
1 tsp turmeric
1 tsp coriander
2 tsp curry powder
1 cup white wine
1/4 cup canola or olive oil
1/2 cup golden raisins
2 cups cooked quinoa
2-3 cups arugula

Dressing:
2 tbl dijon mustard
1/4 cup white wine vinegar
2 tsp paprika
1/2 cup olive oil
salt and pepper

Preparation

Preheat oven to 400˚F.
Whisk the spices in the white wine and oil. Pour over cauliflower, tossing to coat completely, spread out on a sheet pan and cook for about 20 minutes, or until tender.
Make the dressing: whisk together dijon, vinegar and paprika, slowly whisk in olive oil and season with salt and pepper.
When ready to eat toss arugula and quinoa with dressing, add raisins and cauliflower.

Honey Lime Sriracha Glazed Cauliflower Wings

Ingredients

For the sauce:
1/4 cup sriracha
1 Tablespoons soy sauce
1/4 c honey (or maple syrup)
2 Tablespoons lime juice

For the cauliflower:
One large head cauliflower
1/2 c all purpose flour
1/2 c milk of choice
1/2 t garlic powder
Optional scallions for garnish, if desired

Preparation

For the sauce:
Combine all of the sauce ingredients in a bowl and whisk together. Set aside.

For the cauliflower:
Preheat your oven to 450°F, and spray a baking sheet with oil or cooking spray.
Cut the cauliflower into florets. The smaller they are, the faster they will cook and softer they will get.
Whisk together the remaining ingredients in a bowl.
Toss the cauliflower in the batter until thoroughly coated.
Arrange the cauliflower on the baking sheet in a single layer.
Bake for 15-20 minutes, or until slightly less done than you want them.
Remove from the oven and pour the sauce over the cauliflower .
Return to oven for another 5 minutes.
Remove from the oven and gently flip and toss the cauliflower in the sauce on the sheet.
Return to the oven for another 5 minutes.
Place the cauliflower on a serving plate or bowl, and if desired, sprinkle with scallions.

Cauliflower Chowder

Ingredients

4 slices bacon, diced
2 tablespoons unsalted butter
2 cloves garlic, minced
1 onion, diced
2 carrots, peeled and diced
2 stalks celery, diced
1/4 cup all-purpose flour
4 cups chicken broth
1 cup 2% milk
1 head cauliflower, roughly chopped
1 bay leaf
Kosher salt and freshly ground black pepper, to taste
2 tablespoons chopped fresh parsley leaves

Preparation

Heat a large stockpot or Dutch oven over medium heat. Add bacon and cook until brown and crispy, about 6-8 minutes. Transfer to a paper towel-lined plate; set aside.

Melt butter in a large stockpot or Dutch oven over medium heat. Add garlic, onion, carrots and celery. Cook, stirring occasionally, until tender, about 3-4 minutes. Stir in cauliflower and bay leaf. Cook, stirring occasionally, until barely crisp-tender, about 3-4 minutes.

Whisk in flour until lightly browned, about 1 minute. Gradually whisk in chicken broth and milk, and cook, whisking constantly, until slightly thickened, about 3-4 minutes.

Bring to a boil; reduce heat and simmer until cauliflower are tender, about 12-15 minutes; season with salt and pepper, to taste. If the chowder is too thick, add more milk as needed until desired consistency is reached.

Serve immediately, garnished with bacon and parsley, if desired.

Cauliflower Breakfast Muffin

Ingredients

2½ cup finely diced cauliflower (in food processor)
1 Tablespoon ground flaxseed
2 eggs, beaten
1/4 teaspoon salt
pinch pepper
2/3 cup diced lean ham
2 cups grated sharp cheddar cheese or your favorite cheese
2/3 cup diced mushrooms (optional)
12 Jalapeno slices (optional)

Preparation

Preheat oven to 375 degrees.
Place muffin liners in a 12 muffin tin and coat liners with non-stick spray.
In a medium size mixing bowl, combine all ingredients except jalapenoes.
Divide mixture evenly beween muffin liners and place jalapeno slice on top of each muffin (if desired).
Bake for 30 minutes or until golden brown.

Coffee

Calories: zero

Black coffee is one of the lowest-calorie drink choices around, and it's a great weight loss ally. Coffee alters levels of gut peptides, the hormones naturally released to control hunger or fullness.

Coffee drinkers may be at lower risk of liver and colon cancer, type 2 diabetes, and Parkinson's disease, and it may help you live longer: A 2008 study found that women who drank coffee regularly—up to six cups a day—were less likely to die of various causes during the study than their non-coffee-drinking counterparts.

What's more the caffeine in coffee can speed up metabolism and fat-burning, which helps lower your risk of type 2 diabetes and obesity.

Iced Coffee

Ingredients

1/2 cup sugar
1/2 teaspoon vanilla extract
1 cup coffee, at room temperature
2 tablespoons half and half, or more, to taste(Or Milk as you like)

Preparation

To make the simple syrup, combine sugar and 1 cup water in a medium saucepan over medium heat, stirring until the sugar has dissolved. Let cool completely and stir in vanilla extract; set aside.
Serve coffee over ice with half and half and simple syrup, to taste.

Grapefruit

Calories: 39 per half fruit

Remember The Grapefruit Diet? There may be something to that. Studies reveal that, on average, women who consumed any amount of grapefruit or grapefruit juice weighed nearly 10 pounds less and had a 6 percent lower body mass index (BMI) than their non-grapefruit-eating counterparts.

A powerhouse for heart health, grapefruit contains vitamin C, folic acid, and potassium, along with pectin, a soluble fiber that may be a strong ally against atherosclerosis. Pink and red varieties also have vitamin A and lycopene, a phytochemical that protects arterial walls from oxidative damage.

Grapefruit, Walnut, and Feta Salad

Ingredients

1 small red grapefruit
2 tablespoons extra-virgin olive oil
1/2 teaspoon sugar
1/8 teaspoon salt
1/8 teaspoon black pepper
4 cups torn lettuce
4 tablespoons crumbled feta cheese
4 tablespoons toasted walnuts

Preparation

1. Peel and section grapefruit over a bowl; squeeze membranes to extract juice. Set sections aside; reserve 3 tablespoons juice. Discard membranes.

2. Combine juice, olive oil, sugar, salt, and pepper, stirring with a whisk. Put lettuce in a bow, sprinkle crumbled feta cheese and toasted walnuts over it. Add grapefruit and drizzle with vinaigrette.

Avocado Cucumber Grapefruit Salad

Ingredients

Salad
2 cucumbers, diced, seeds removed
3-4 grapefruit or oranges, peeled and chopped
2-3 avocados, diced (about 1½ cups)
1/3 cup almonds, chopped
2 tablespoons fresh mint, chopped
3-4 tablespoons fresh chives, chopped

Dressing
1 tablespoon vinegar (can also use lime or lemon juice)
1½ tablespoon honey
1½ tablespoons olive oil
salt to taste
grapefruit or orange zest to taste

Preparation

Wash, cut, and gently toss the cucumbers, grapefruit, almonds, mint, and chives.
Whisk the dressing ingredients together. Taste and adjust to your preferences. Drizzle over the salad ingredients. Chill until ready to serve.
Just before serving, gently mix the avocado pieces into the salad. Top with additional herbs or almonds.

Grapefruit Spinach Salad Recipe

Ingredients

1 medium pink grapefruit
1 package (10 ounces) fresh spinach, torn
2 tablespoons chopped green onion
2 teaspoons cider vinegar
2 teaspoons olive oil
2 teaspoons honey
2 teaspoons prepared mustard

Preparation

Cut grapefruit in half; with a sharp knife, cut around each section to loosen fruit, reserving juice. In a salad bowl, toss the spinach, onion and grapefruit sections. In a jar with a tight-fitting lid, combine the vinegar, oil, honey, mustard and reserved grapefruit juice; shake well. Drizzle over salad and toss to coat. Serve immediately.

Mushrooms

Calories: 15 per cup

Meaty and incredibly low-cal, mushrooms are also incredibly diverse. White button, Portobello, shiitake, and Maitake are just a few of the varieties you'll find in your grocery store. Fortunately, just about all mushrooms contain some form of immune-boosting antioxidants, along with potassium, B vitamins, and fiber.

Shiitakes, for example, contain lentinan, a nutrient that is thought to have anticancer properties. All mushrooms are good sources of vitamin D, thiamin, riboflavin, niacin, vitamin B6, pantothenic acid, phosphorus, potassium, copper and selenium.

Stuffed Masala Mushrooms

Ingredients

For the stuffing:
1 tsp oil
2 tsp butter
1 tsp cumin
1 chopped Kashmiri chilli
1 large onion, chopped
1 tsp chopped garlic
1 tsp red chilli powder
1 tsp coriander seeds
Salt, to taste
Water, to deglaze
1 tomato chopped
1 cup corn kernels
Sugar, a pinch
10 mushroom stalks, chopped
Parsley, chopped

For the mushroom caps:
10 mushroom caps
1 tsp butter
Sea salt, to sprinkle
Pepper, to sprinkle
Mozzarella cheese, grated
Coriander leaves, to garnish

Preparation

For the stuffing:
In a pan add 1 tsp oil and 2 tsp butter.
Add cumin, Kashmiri chilli. Saute.
Add onions and saute till brown.   Add garlic, red chilli powder, coriander, salt. Saute and add some water to de glaze.
Now add the tomatoes. Saute and add a pinch of sugar to balance acidity.
Add corn. Cook till the tomato and corn are cooked.
Add the chopped 10 mushroom stalks. Cook till the mushrooms leave some water of their own and that water dries up.
Add some chopped parsley. Mix and keep aside.

For the mushroom caps:

In a baking tray arrange mushroom caps which are properly washed and the stalks are removed.

In the mushroom cavity add a little butter, sprinkle some sea salt and pepper.

Add the stuffing generously.

Grate some cheese over them. Keep aside for 5-7 minutes.

Bake at 180 degrees for 15 minutes.

Garnish with coriander leaves.

Serve with a dipping sauce of your choice.

Mushroom Pasta

Ingredients

12 oz rigatoni
1¼ lb mushrooms, sliced
1 onion, chopped
1 tsp dried thyme
1 tsp minced garlic
3/4 c white wine
1 c reduced-sodium chicken broth
3 Tbsp mascarpone
Parmesan
Parsley

Preparation

Cook rigatoni.
Heat oil in large nonstick skillet over medium-high heat. Add mushrooms, onion, thyme, and garlic. Cook until golden, 7 minutes. Add wine and reduce by half. Stir in broth and mascarpone. Toss with pasta, Parmesan, and parsley.

Cream of Mushroom & Barley Soup

Ingredients

1/2 cup pearl barley
4 1/2 cups reduced-sodium chicken broth, or mushroom broth
1 ounce dried porcini mushrooms
2 cups boiling water
2 teaspoons butter
1 tablespoon extra-virgin olive oil
1 cup minced shallots
8 cups sliced white mushrooms, (about 20 ounces)
2 stalks celery, finely chopped
1 tablespoon minced fresh sage, or 1 teaspoon dried
1/2 teaspoon salt
1/2 teaspoon freshly ground pepper
2 tablespoons all-purpose flour
1 cup dry sherry
1/2 cup reduced-fat sour cream
1/4 cup minced fresh chives

Preparation

Bring barley and 1 1/2 cups broth to a boil in a small saucepan over high heat. Cover, reduce heat to low and simmer until tender, 30 to 35 minutes.

Meanwhile, combine porcinis and boiling water in a medium bowl and soak until softened, about 20 minutes. Line a sieve with paper towels, set it over a bowl and pour in mushrooms and soaking liquid. Reserve the soaking liquid. Transfer the mushrooms to a cutting board and finely chop.

Heat butter and oil in a Dutch oven over medium-high heat. Add shallots and cook, stirring often, until softened, about 2 minutes. Add white mushrooms and cook, stirring often, until they start to brown, 8 to 10 minutes. Add the porcinis, celery, sage, salt and pepper and cook, stirring often, until beginning to soften, about 3 minutes. Sprinkle flour over the vegetables and cook, stirring, until the flour is incorporated, about 1 minute. Add sherry and cook, stirring, until most of the sherry has evaporated, about 1 minute.

Add the soaking liquid and the remaining 3 cups broth; increase heat to high and bring to a boil. Reduce heat and simmer, stirring occasionally, until the soup has thickened, 18 to 22 minutes.

Add the cooked barley and continue cooking, stirring occasionally, until heated through, about 5 minutes more. Stir in sour cream until incorporated. Garnish with chives.

Tomatoes

Calories: 22 per medium tomato

They contain lycopene, an antioxidant rarely found in other foods. Studies suggest that it could protect the skin against harmful UV rays, prevent certain cancers, and lower cholesterol. Plus, tomatoes contain high amounts of potassium, fiber, and vitamin C.

Tomato Salad with Edamame

Ingredients

3 tablespoons olive oil
1/4 teaspoon crushed red pepper
2 cups frozen sweet edamame, thawed
2 cups fresh corn kernels or 2 cups frozen whole kernel corn, thawed
3/4 cup chopped red sweet pepper
1/2 cup sliced green onion
2 tablespoons freshly squeezed lemon juice
2 tablespoons snipped fresh flat-leaf Italian parsley
2 tablespoons snipped fresh mint
1/2 teaspoon salt, divided
3 pounds medium to large heirloom tomatoes, cored and sliced 1/4-inch thick
1/4 teaspoon ground black pepper

Preparation

Heat oil and crushed red pepper in a large skillet over medium-high heat for 1 minute. Add edamame, corn and red sweet pepper. Cook and stir for 4 minutes. Add green onion; cook and stir for 3 to 4 minutes or until vegetables are tender. Add lemon juice, parsley, mint and 1/4 teaspoon salt. Stir to combine; remove from heat.

Arrange tomato slices on salad plates or a platter. Sprinkle with remaining 1/4 teaspoon salt. Spoon warm vegetables over tomatoes. Sprinkle with black pepper.

Tropical Tomato Salsa

Ingredients

3 medium yellow and/or red tomatoes, seeded and chopped
1 cup chopped seedless watermelon
1 medium mango, halved, seeded, peeled and chopped
1/3 cup finely chopped red onion
1/4 cup snipped fresh cilantro
2 jalapeno peppers, halved, seeded and finely chopped
3 tablespoons lime juice
2 teaspoons honey
Kosher salt

Preparation

In a medium bowl combine tomatoes, watermelon, mango, red onion, cilantro, jalapeno, lime juice, and honey. Stir gently to combine. Season to taste with kosher salt. Cover and chill until ready to serve.

Roasted Tomato Basil Pesto Pasta

Ingredients

large roma tomatoes, sliced in half lengthwise
1/2 cup almonds, toasted
2 garlic cloves
1 cup tightly packed basil + more for garnish
1/4 cup extra virgin olive oil + more for drizzling on tomatoes
salt & black pepper, to taste
Your desired amount of cooked Pasta

Preparation

1. Preheat oven to 400F and line a baking sheet with parchment. Place sliced tomatoes on the sheet and drizzle with oil, salt, and pepper. Roast for about 1 hour and 10 mins at 400F. Watch closely during the last 15 minutes of roasting.

2. Reduce oven heat to 325F and toast almonds for 8-10 minutes. Add 1/3 cup into food processor and process until finely chopped. I left mine a bit chunky for texture. Remove and set aside.

3. With processor turned on, add 2 garlic cloves and let it whirl around until finely chopped. Now add in the basil and process until finely chopped.

4. Add in the oil, and 1.5 cups of roasted tomatoes (you will have tomatoes left over). Process until smooth. Pulse in 1/3 cup toasted almonds. Season generously with salt and pepper.

5. Pour your desired amount of pesto over the cooked pasta and mix well. Chop the remaining roasted tomatoes and stir into pasta.

Zucchini

Calories: 20 per cup

This miracle squash is the ultimate high volume food, meaning you can fill up on very few calories. It's easy to grow, especially in the summer, packs lots of vitamin A, and is so simple to prepare raw or cook with you may want to eat it all year!

Sautéed Zucchini

Ingredients

1 medium unpeeled garlic clove
2 teaspoons extra-virgin olive oil
1/4 teaspoon red pepper flakes
1 pound zucchini (about 4 medium), trimmed and cut into 2-by-1/4-inch matchsticks
Salt and ground black pepper
2 tablespoons finely grated Parmesan cheese

Preparation

Smash the garlic clove by pushing on the knife blade with the heel of your hand. Remove and discard the peel and set the garlic clove aside.

Heat the oil in a large frying pan over medium-high heat until shimmering. Add the garlic and red pepper flakes and cook, stirring occasionally, until fragrant but not browned, about 30 seconds.
Remove the garlic with a slotted spoon or tongs and discard (or save for another use).

Add the zucchini to the pan and toss until coated with oil. Let cook undisturbed until the bottoms of the matchsticks are golden brown, about 1 minute. Toss again and cook until crisp-tender, about 1 minute more. Remove the pan from heat and season the zucchini with salt and pepper.

Transfer the zucchini to a serving dish and sprinkle with the Parmesan. Serve immediately.

Ratatouille

Ingredients

1/3 cup olive oil, divided
1 medium eggplant, sliced into ¾-in.-thick rounds
1½ tsp salt
1 small Spanish onion, chopped (about 2 cups)
1 green pepper, diced (about 1½ cups)
1 red pepper, diced (about 1½ cups)
3 small zucchini or summer squash, cut into ¾-in. cubes (about 4 cups)
2 tbsp chopped garlic
1 28-oz can Italian plum tomatoes, diced (or about 2 lb. peeled, chopped tomatoes)
1/4 cup basil leaves, torn
pinch of sugar

Preparation

Preheat oven to 450F.

Use 3 tbsp of olive oil to brush eggplant on both sides. Season with ¼ tsp salt. Place in a single layer on a baking sheet and bake for 20 min, turning after 15 min or until tender and lightly browned. Let cool. Dice and reserve.

Heat remaining 3 tbsp oil in a dutch oven or large, heavy-bottomed pot. Add onions and sauté over medium heat for 4 min or until soft. Add peppers and sauté for 4 min or until softened. 4. Add zucchini, garlic and ½ tsp salt and sauté for 4 min longer or until softened. Add tomatoes and basil, cover and bring to a simmer for 20 min or until vegetables are soft.

Add eggplant, remaining ¾ tsp salt and pinch of sugar and simmer for 5 min longer or until flavours have combined.

Serve with crusty bread or over 250 g buttered tagliatelle pasta, cooked according to package directions.

Coconut Chickpea Curry

Ingredients

2 tbsp canola oil
1 cup chopped red onion
2 tbsp chopped ginger
1 tbsp chopped garlic
4 tsp Madras curry paste
2 cups canned tomatoes (from a drained 796-mL can), mashed
1 400-mL can light coconut milk
¼ cup water
3 cups diced sweet potato (about ¾-in. dice)
3 cups Not-Canned Chickpeas
2 cups diced zucchini
1 tsp salt
3 tbsp chopped coriander

Preparation

Heat canola oil in a wide pot over medium. Add onion and sauté for 4 min or until so! ened. Add ginger, garlic and curry paste, and sauté for 1 min longer. Add tomatoes, coconut milk and water, and bring to a boil.

Add sweet potatoes, turn heat to medium-low and simmer for 15 min or until sweet potatoes are tender but not soft.

Add chickpeas and zucchini, and simmer for 15 min longer or until zucchini is soft. Season with salt and sprinkle with chopped coriander. Serve over rice or with a side of toasted naan.

Spinach

Calories: 7 per cup

Tender and flavorful, this leafy green is rich in iron, folic acid, and vitamin K. It also contains disease-fighting antioxidants beta-carotene and vitamin C, as well as the phytochemical lutein, which protects eyes against age-related macular degeneration.

Fresh Spinach Dip

Ingredients

2 tablespoons olive oil
1 medium carrot, finely chopped
1/2 cup yellow onion, small dice
2 medium garlic cloves, finely chopped
1 teaspoon kosher salt, plus more as needed
1/2 teaspoon freshly ground black pepper, plus more as needed
20 ounces baby spinach, washed
2 medium scallions, finely chopped (white and light green parts only)
1 cup sour cream
1/2 cup mayonnaise
2 teaspoons Worcestershire sauce
1 teaspoon freshly squeezed lemon juice
Saltine or Ritz crackers, crostini, carrot sticks, celery sticks, or thick-cut potato chips, for serving

Preparation

Place a quadruple layer of paper towels on a cutting board and set aside. Place a fine-mesh strainer in the sink.

Heat the oil in a large straight-sided frying pan over medium heat until shimmering. Add the carrot, onion, garlic, measured salt, and measured pepper and stir to combine. Cook, stirring occasionally, until the vegetables have softened, about 6 minutes. Transfer to a large bowl and set aside.

Return the pan to medium heat, add half of the spinach, season with salt and pepper, and stir to combine. Cook, tossing occasionally with tongs, until the spinach is completely wilted, about 4 minutes. Add the remaining spinach and cook, tossing occasionally, until completely wilted, about 3 minutes more.

Transfer the spinach to the strainer in the sink. Using a ladle, press on the spinach to squeeze out as much liquid as possible.

Place the spinach on the layered paper towels, cover with a second quadruple layer of paper towels, and press any additional liquid out of the leaves. Discard the paper towels, finely chop the spinach, and transfer it to the bowl with the vegetables.

Add the scallions, sour cream, mayonnaise, Worcestershire, and lemon juice and stir to combine. Cover tightly and refrigerate until the flavors meld and the dip is thoroughly chilled, about 2 hours.

Taste and season with salt and pepper as needed, then transfer to a serving dish. Serve with saltine or Ritz crackers, crostini, carrot sticks, celery sticks, or thick-cut potato chips.

Strawberry Spinach Salad

Ingredients

For dressing:
2 tbsp worcestershire sauce
2 tbsp white vinegar
1/4 cup vegetable oil
3 tbsp granulated sugar
1/2 tbsp finely grated onion
1 tbsp poppy seeds
Salt to taste

For Salad:
12 cups (2-10 oz bags) baby spinach
2 cups (1 pint) strawberries, hulled and sliced
1/2 cup sliced almonds, toasted
4 oz (6 tbsp/110 g) soft goat cheese or feta, crumbled

Preparation

Whisk together all dressing ingredients, taste, and add more salt if needed.

In a large bowl, combine baby spinach and sliced strawberries. Add a splash of dressing and toss. Repeat, adding small amounts of dressing and tossing until leaves are lightly coated (you will have extra dressing).

Divide among six plates and top with sliced almonds and goat cheese (or add almonds and cheese to the large bowl and gently toss everything together).

Spinach Soup

Ingredients

2 1/2 qt stock
1 carrot
1 celery stalk
a few celery leaves
salt and pepper to taste
2 tbsp flour
2 tbsp butter
3 egg yolks
1 lemon

Preparation

If using fresh spinach, wash and place in a pan over low heat and cover. When they collapse into a soft mass, chop.

Put stock, carrot and celery in a pan. Bring to a boil and season to taste with salt and pepper. Simmer 20 minutes until carrots are tender.

In a small pan, melt butter and when frothy, add flour to make a rue. When light golden in color, whisk in a ladleful of the soup and add gradually to the pot of stock. Simmer over low heat for another 10 minutes, then stir in spinach and simmer 10 minutes more.

Beat egg yolks and lemon juice together in a bowl. Add a ladleful of the soup to the egg yolk mixture to temper, then pour into the soup slowing stirring constantly. This will add a lovely velvety texture to the soup that is without parallel. Do not allow the soup to come back to a boil or you will loose this texture. Serve immediately.

Lemons and limes

Calories: 20 per fruit (without peel)

Citrus fruits are loaded with vitamin C and, eaten whole, are a great source of fiber. Studies show that loading up on C-rich citrus at the first sign of illness may reduce a cold's duration by about a day. We also love adding a splash of lemon or lime juice to recipes.

Often tart and sometimes sweet citrus flavors add a punch of flavor without any added fat, calories, or cholesterol.

Lime soda

Ingredients

2 tablespoons simple syrup (made by first boiling together equal parts sugar and water, then letting it cool)
1 1/2 tablespoon freshly squeezed lime juice (regular supermarket limes are the best ones to use)
3/4 cup soda water
lime slice

Preparation

Fill a glass with ice cubes, then add simple syrup and lime juice. Add soda water. Stir well, then serve garnished with a lime slice, if you like.

Healthy Baked Lemon Chicken

Ingredients

4 boneless skinless chicken breasts
3 tablespoons butter
⅓ cup chicken broth
4 tablespoons fresh lemon juice
1 tablespoon honey
2 teaspoons minced garlic
1 teaspoon Italian seasoning
salt and pepper to taste
optional: fresh rosemary and lemon slices for garnish

Preparation

Preheat oven to 400 degrees and grease a baking sheet or large casserole dish.

Melt butter in a large skillet over medium-high heat. Add chicken and cook chicken 2-3 minutes on each side just until browned. Transfer chicken to prepared baking sheet.

In a small bowl whisk together chicken broth, lemon juice, honey, garlic, Italian seasoning, and salt and pepper.

Pour sauce over chicken. Bake 20-30 minutes (closer to 20 for smaller chicken breasts, closer to 30 for larger) until chicken is cooked through. Every 5-10 minutes spoon the sauce from the pan over the chicken.

Garnish with fresh rosemary and lemon slices if desired and serve.

Lemon Bars

Ingredients

For Base
2 cups sifted flour
1⁄2 cup powdered sugar
1 cup butter

For top
4 large beaten eggs
2 cups white sugar
1⁄3 cup lemon juice
1⁄4 cup flour
1⁄2 teaspoon baking powder
1⁄2 teaspoon fresh lemon rind (optional)

Preparation

For the base mix the butter into the flour and sugar.
Mix with hands until it clings together.
Press into a 13 x 9 x 2-inch pan.
Bake at 350°F for 20-25 minutes or until lightly browned.
For the filling, beat together eggs, sugar and lemon juice.
Sift together flour and baking powder.
Stir into egg mixture.
Pour over baked, cooled crust.
Bake at 350°F for 25 minutes.
Cool and sprinkle with powdered sugar.
Cut into bars.

Kale

Calories: 5 per cup

Kale is possibly the healthiest superfood around, packing a widevariety of phytonutrients that may prevent cancer, including breast cancer. (Scientsits theorize that the phytonutrients in kale trigger the liver to produce enzymes that neutralize potentially cancer-causing substances.)

Kale is also a great source of B vitamins, folic acid, and manganese, which helps regulate blood sugar and is essential for proper immune system function.

Kale With Roasted Peppers and Olives

Ingredients

2 large bunches kale
2tablespoons olive oil
2 cloves garlic, thinly sliced
2teaspoons sugar
1teaspoon salt
12 olives, pitted and chopped
1 4-ounce jar roasted red peppers
2tablespoons aged balsamic vinegar

Preparation

Cut the kale into bite-size pieces, removing any tough stems. Rinse and shake dry.
Warm the oil and garlic in a large stockpot over medium-high heat. Remove the garlic
as soon as it browns (don't let it burn). Add the kale and stir-fry 5 minutes. Add 1/4
cup water, cover, and cook 8 to 10 minutes or until tender. Uncover and add the sugar,
salt, olives, and peppers. Cook over medium-high heat until the liquid has evaporated.
Spoon into a serving dish; scatter the garlic over the top. Drizzle with the balsamic
vinegar. Serve warm or at room temperature.

Vegetable Barley Soup

Ingredients

1 1/2 cups barley
1/4cup olive oil
6 carrots, diced
6 stalks celery, diced
4 large onions, diced
4 parsnips, diced
salt and black pepper
1 102-ounce can diced tomatoes (or four 28-ounce cans)
1 bunch kale, thick stems discarded and leaves chopped (about 8 cups)
2 15.5-ounce cans chickpeas, rinsed

Preparation

Cook the barley according to the package directions.

Meanwhile, heat the oil in a large pot or Dutch oven. Add the carrots, celery, onions, parsnips, 1 teaspoon salt, and 1/2 teaspoon pepper. Cook, covered, stirring occasionally, until the vegetables begin to soften, 20 to 25 minutes.

Add the tomatoes (and their juices) and 8 cups water. Simmer, stirring occasionally, until the soup has slightly thickened and the vegetables are tender, 45 to 60 minutes.

Add the kale and simmer, stirring occasionally, until it is tender, 5 to 6 minutes. Stir in the chickpeas and cooked barley and cook until heated through, about 3 minutes.

Kale Smoothie

Ingredients

3/4cup chopped kale, ribs and thick stems removed
1 small stalk celery, chopped
1/2 banana
1/2cup apple juice
1/2cup ice
1tablespoon fresh lemon juice

Preparation

Place the kale, celery, banana, apple juice, ice, and lemon juice in a blender.
Blend until smooth and frothy.

Garlic

Calories: 4 per clove

Garlic fights colds, battles cancer, and may even ward off urinary tract infections. A diet rich in garlic can help thanks to the bulb's natural antimicrobial properties.

To get the most health benefits out of this stinky bulb, let chopped or crushed garlic sit for 10 minutes before heating. This method helps it retain a third more of its cancer-fighting sulfur compounds than if it were cooked immediately.

Garlic & Herb Yogurt Dip

Ingredients

3/4 cup plain Greek-style low-fat yogurt
1 garlic clove, minced
2 tablespoons chopped chives
1/4 teaspoon salt
1/4 teaspoon pepper
1/4 teaspoon dried dill
1 tablespoon lemon juice
4 ounces baked potato chips

Preparation

Combine first 7 ingredients in a small bowl. Serve with chips.

Garlic Bread

Ingredients

2 teaspoons finely chopped garlic
1/2 stick (1/4 cup) unsalted butter, softened
1 tablespoon extra-virgin olive oil
2 tablespoons finely chopped fresh flat-leaf parsley
1 (15- by 3 1/2-inch) loaf Italian bread

Preparation

Preheat oven to 350°F.

Mince and mash garlic to a paste with a rounded 1/4 teaspoon salt using a heavy knife. Stir together butter, oil, and garlic paste in a bowl until smooth, then stir in parsley.

Without cutting completely through bottom, cut bread diagonally into 1-inch-thick slices with a serrated knife, then spread garlic butter between slices.

Wrap loaf in foil and bake in middle of oven 15 minutes. Open foil and bake 5 minutes more.

Bread can be spread with garlic butter 8 hours ahead and chilled, wrapped in foil. Let stand at room temperature 30 minutes before baking.

Mussels with Garlic

Ingredients

4 cloves garlic
Kosher salt
4 tbsp. chopped flat-leaf parsley, plus 1⁄4 cup leaves
6 anchovies, chopped
2 tbsp. olive oil
2 cups white wine
3 lb. mussels, debearded
Zest of 1 lemon

Preparation

Make a paste with the garlic and a little salt. Top garlic with chopped parsley and anchovies; chop together to form a smooth paste.

Heat oil in a 6-qt. pot over medium-high heat. Add paste; cook, stirring, until aromatic, about 2 minutes. Add wine; boil for 2 minutes. Add mussels; cover and steam until they open, 3-4 minutes. Sprinkle mussels with parsley leaves and zest. Toss with a spoon. Serve mussels and broth in bowls with crusty bread to sop up the savory liquid.

Peppers

Calories: 30 per half cup

Hot or mild, peppers are packed with vitamin C fiber for negligible calories. The heat in hot peppers signals the presence of capsaicin, a compound that, along with capsiate, can propel the body to scorch an extra 50 to 100 calories following a spicy meal.

Baked Eggs in Stuffed Peppers with Butternut Squash Hash

Ingredients

3 sweet bell peppers, red, orange or yellow
2 tablespoons butter
1 tablespoon olive oil
2 cloves garlic, diced
½ cup onion, chopped
1 pound butternut squash, peeled, seeded and cut into a large dice, about 2 cups
1 teaspoon dried thyme leaves
Kosher salt
1/4 cup brandy
1/2 cup Ricotta cheese
1/4 cup crumbled Feta cheese
6 eggs
2 cups prepared marinara sauce
Freshly ground black pepper

Preparation

Preheat oven to 400 F°.

Cut peppers in half and remove ribs and seeds. Place cut side up in shallow microwave safe bowl or dish. Add ⅓ cup water to bowl. Sprinkle peppers with kosher salt and cover with plastic wrap. Microwave on high for 5 minutes. Remove and set aside.

Heat large skillet over medium high heat and melt butter and olive oil. Add garlic and cook for 1 minute, stirring after 30 seconds. Add onion and sauté for 2-3 minutes, stirring occasionally. Add butternut squash, thyme leaves and kosher salt and cook for another 5 minutes. Remove from heat. Add brandy. Return to heat and cook for 4-5 more minutes until brandy has cooked down and squash has softened and is easily pierced with a fork. Keep warm and add Ricotta and Feta cheese. Taste and season with more salt if desired.

Pour marinara sauce in bottom of 9 x 12 inch baking dish. Place peppers cut side up and spoon ½ to ¾ cup of butternut squash mixture into each pepper, creating a hollow for egg. Bake peppers and squash mixture for 10 minutes or until warmed through. Remove from oven.

Carefully break egg into small ramekin or measuring cup and slowly pour into each pepper taking care not to overflow egg. Repeat until each pepper is filled.

Season with freshly ground black pepper and bake peppers for 10-12 minutes or until whites of eggs are set. Serve each pepper with marinara sauce and extra feta cheese if desired.

Spicy Red Pepper Sauce

Ingredients

2 whole roasted red peppers, seeds removed
2 dried ancho chilies
1 dried chile de arbol
2 chipotle chiles in adobo
1 cup boiling water
1 garlic clove, peeled + smashed
Juice of half a lemon
Salt, to taste
2 tablespoons olive oil

Preparation

Place the dried chiles in a heatproof bowl and pour the boiling water over top the chiles. Let sit for 20 to 30 minutes until the chiles are softened. Reserve chile water. Once chiles are softened, cut top off the chiles and remove the seeds from inside. Add to the bowl of a food processor or blender, along with the chipotle chiles in adobo, garlic and lemon juice. Purée, slowly pouring in the olive oil to thicken the sauce. If desired add 1-2 tablespoons of the reserved chile water to thin the sauce a bit. Season to taste with salt and extra lemon juice. It will keep refrigerated for a few weeks.

Spicy Sausage And Pepper Pasta

Ingredients

12 ounces Penne pasta
2 tablespoons olive oil
1/2 red onion, sliced
2 cloves garlic, minced
1/2 red bell pepper, cut into strips
1/2 orange bell pepper, cut into strips
1/2 yellow bell pepper, cut into strips
1 package Butterball Turkey Sausage (13 oz), cut into 1/2 inch rounds
Crushed red pepper, to taste
1 1/2 cups grape tomatoes, halved
1 cup shredded Parmesan cheese
1/3 cup chopped fresh basil
Salt and black pepper, to taste

Preparation

1. In a large pot of boiling salted water, cook pasta until al dente.

2. While the pasta is cooking, heat the olive oil over medium-high heat in a large sauté pan. Add the onion, garlic, peppers, and sausage. Cook for about 5 minutes, stirring occasionally.

3. Drain the pasta and pour into a large serving bowl. Stir in the onions, peppers, and sausage. Add the tomatoes, Parmesan cheese, and basil. Season with salt and black pepper, to taste. Serve immediately.

Onions

Calories: 32 per half cup

Don't hold the onions! These flavorful bulbs, which range from sweet to sharp in flavor, boast allyl sulfides, compounds that have been shown to protect against endometrial cancer in laboratory studies.

French onion soup

Ingredients

2 tablespoons olive oil
2 onions, thinly sliced
2 fresh thyme sprigs
2 tablespoons plain flour
1/2 cup sweet sherry
6 cups salt-reduced chicken stock
30cm baguette
cooking spray
100g cheese, grated

Preparation

Heat oil in a large, heavy-based saucepan over medium-low heat. Add onion and thyme. Cook, stirring often, for 45 minutes or until onion is browned and softened.

Increase heat to medium. Add flour. Cook, stirring, for 2 minutes. Add sherry. Cook, stirring, for 2 minutes or until bubbling. Add stock and 2 cups cold water. Cover. Bring to the boil. Reduce heat to low. Simmer for 20 minutes or until slightly thickened.

Meanwhile, preheat oven to 200°C/180°C fan-forced. Cut eight 1.5cm slices from bread. Spray both sides bread with oil. Place on a baking tray. Bake, turning once, for 5 minutes or until lightly browned. Top with cheese. Bake for 2 to 3 minutes or until cheese has melted.

Ladle soup into bowls. Top each with 1 cheese toast. Season with salt and pepper. Serve with remaining cheese toast.

Tomato, red onion and balsamic salsa

Ingredients

2 1/2 tablespoons extra-virgin olive oil
1 garlic clove, crushed
1 tablespoon balsamic vinegar
500g grape or mini roma tomatoes, roughly chopped
1 small red onion, finely diced
1/4 cup flat-leaf parsley leaves, chopped
Salt and pepper

Preparation

Place oil, garlic and vinegar in a bowl. Add tomatoes, onion and parsley. Season with salt and pepper and stir to combine. Stand for 10 minutes. Serve with barbecued steak or lamb kebabs.

Glazed onions

Ingredients

6 yellow onions, unpeeled
1 tablespoon olive oil
1 tablespoon balsamic vinegar
2 tablespoons sugar
1/4 cup Vegetable Stock
5 sprigs fresh thyme leaves
2 green onions, thinly sliced

Preparation

Cut onions in half lengthways. Remove skin. Trim ends, leaving base intact

Heat oil in a frying pan over medium heat. Cook onion, turning, for 3 to 5 minutes or until golden. Add vinegar and sugar. Cook for 2 minutes. Add stock and thyme. Cook, covered, brushing with vinegar mixture, for 5 to 7 minutes or until tender. Add green onion. Toss to combine. Serve.

Pumpkin

Calories: 30 per cup

This low-calorie squash is rich in potassium and loaded with beta-carotene (a powerful antioxidant), and its natural sweetness brings flavor to baked goods without any added guilt. It's a great source of vitamins A, C, and E, and packs potassium (great for lowering blood pressure) and copper.

Eating pumpkin may even be good for diabetes; studies found two compounds in this vegetable, trigonelline and nicotinic acid, improved glucose tolerance in rats.

Coconut Curry Pumpkin Soup

Ingredients

2 tbsp. extra-virgin olive oil
1 small onion, finely chopped
1 clove garlic, minced
2 tsp. fresh ginger, grated
2 tsp. curry powder
1 1/2 tsp. cinnamon
1 tsp. nutmeg
1/2 tsp. cloves
Salt and pepper
3 c. pumpkin puree (fresh or canned)
1/4 c. brown sugar, packed
4 c. vegetable (or chicken) stock
1 14-oz. can coconut milk
Toasted pumpkin seeds, for garnish
Cilantro leaves, for garnish

Preparation

Heat oil in large pot over medium-high heat. Add onion and cook until tender, 4 to 5 minutes. Add garlic and ginger, stirring, until fragrant, 1 minute. Stir in curry, cinnamon, nutmeg, and cloves and season with salt and pepper.

Stir in pumpkin puree and brown sugar. Whisk in vegetable stock and bring to boil. Reduce heat and simmer until slightly thickened, about 15 minutes. Add coconut milk, cooking over low heat, until warmed through. Season with salt and pepper.

Serve in bowls and garnish with toasted pumpkin seeds and cilantro.

Pumpkin Biscuits

Ingredients

1½ cups all purpose flour
2 tsp baking powder
1/2 tsp baking soda
1/2 tsp salt
3 tsp dried crumbled sage
2 tbsp cold butter, cut into small pieces
3/4 cup pumpkin puree
1/2 cup Greek yogurt
2 tbsp butter, melted
10 fresh sage leaves {optional}

Preparation

Pre-heat oven to 425°F. Line two baking sheets with parchment paper and set aside.

In a large bowl, combine flour, baking soda, baking powder, salt and sage.

Cut in the butter, blending with a fork or pastry blender until butter is in small, pea-sized pieces.

In a separate medium bowl, combine the pumpkin puree and Greek yogurt. Mix the greek yogurt/pumpkin mixture into the dried ingredients. You may need to use your hands to get it completely blended.

Knead dough out onto a floured surface 6 or so times. Pat or roll out to a thickness of 0.5 inches. It's easier to pat since the dough is a bit sticky. Cut out circles of 2-3 inches in diameter {I used a glass}.

Transfer circles to baking sheets, brush the tops with melted butter, and place a sage leaf on each biscuit. Bake for 11-14 minutes, until biscuits are firm to the touch and cooked through.

Cool slightly and serve.

Pumpkin-Apple Butter

Ingredients

2 can 100% pure pumpkin
2 c. Applesauce
⅔ c. packed light-brown sugar
1½ tbsp. grated fresh ginger
1 tsp. ground cinnamon
1 tsp. nutmeg

Preparation

Stir all ingredients in a heavy, medium saucepan until blended. Bring to a boil, stirring often.
Reduce heat to low and simmer uncovered, stirring often to prevent scorching, 30 minutes, or until mixture is very thick.

Radishes

Calories: 19 per cup

These brightly colored vegetables are packed with potassium, folic acid, antioxidants, and sulfur compounds that aid in digestion.

Don't forget the leafy green tops, which contain six times the vitamin C and more calcium than the roots. Thinly slice and toss in a fresh green salad or julienne for coleslaw.

Indian Spiced Radishes & Pumpkin

Ingredients

800g pumpkin or squash, cut into small chunks
3 tbsp nut oil
1/2 tsp dried chilli flakes
1/2 tsp turmeric
1/2 tsp cumin
1/2 tsp mustard seeds
2 curry leaves
1 garlic clove, minced or finely grated
1 onion, finely diced
20 radishes, sliced into thick rounds
2 tomatoes, chopped

Preparation

Boil the pumpkin in water for 8-10 minutes until tender. Drain and set aside.
In a large frying pan heat the oil and add the chilli, turmeric, cumin, mustard seeds and curry leaves and cook for a minute or two until they are fragrant but not burnt. Add the garlic and cook for a further 30 seconds.
Add the onions and sauté for a minute then add the radishes and finally the pumpkin.
Season with a good pinch of salt and cook until the vegetables are tender but start to crisp on the outside.
Stir through the chopped tomatoes and serve with chapattis.

Roasted Radishes

Ingredients

2 bunches medium radishes (such as red, pink, and purple; about 20)
1 1/2 tablespoons olive oil
Coarse kosher salt
2 tablespoons (1/4 stick) unsalted butter
1 teaspoon fresh lemon juice

Preparation

Preheat oven to 450°F. Brush large heavy-duty rimmed baking sheet with olive oil. Cut off all but 1/2 inch of green radish tops; reserve trimmed tops and rinse them well, checking for grit. Coarsely chop radish tops and set aside. Cut radishes lengthwise in half and place in medium bowl. Add 1 1/2 tablespoons olive oil and toss thoroughly to coat. Place radishes, cut side down, on prepared baking sheet; sprinkle lightly with coarse salt. Roast until radishes are crisp-tender, stirring occasionally, about 18 minutes. Season to taste with more coarse kosher salt, if desired.

Melt butter in heavy small skillet over medium-high heat. Add pinch of coarse kosher salt to skillet and cook until butter browns, swirling skillet frequently to keep butter solids from burning, about 3 minutes. Remove skillet from heat and stir in fresh lemon juice.

Transfer roasted radishes to warmed shallow serving bowl and drizzle brown butter over. Sprinkle with chopped radish tops and serve.

Fennel

Calories: 27 per cup

This incredibly crunchy, delicious, licorice-flavored veggie freshens your breath, soothes winter coughs, and even flattens your belly. It is also a good source of fiber and contains several vitamins and minerals. We love it raw!

Roasted Squash, Onion And Fennel Toss

Ingredients

1 butternut squash peeled
1 fennel bulb trimmed (or 6 tender stalks of celery)
1 red onion
2 tablespoons olive oil
1 teaspoon herbes de Provence
1/2 teaspoon salt
1/4 teaspoon pepper

Preparation

Halve squash and remove seeds. Remove tough outer leaves from fennel; halve lengthwise and remove core. Cut squash and fennel into 1/2-inch (4 cm) chunks; place in large bowl. Cut onion lengthwise into thin wedges; add to bowl. (Make-ahead: Cover and refrigerate for up to 1 day.)

Add oil, herbes de Provence, salt and pepper to bowl; toss to combine. Spread on greased foil-lined baking sheet. Bake in 425°F (220°C) oven for 45 to 60 minutes or until lightly browned and tender.

Apple Fennel Celery Salad

Ingredients

1/2 cup thinly sliced fennel
1/2 cup sliced celery
1/2 cup red seedless grape halved
1 Red Delicious apple peeled, cored and chopped
1/4 cup toasted chopped walnut

Dressing:
1/4 cup Balkan-style plain yogurt
1 tablespoon liquid honey
2 teaspoons lemon juice
1/2 teaspoon Dijon mustard
1/4 teaspoon poppy seeds
1 pinch salt
1 pinch paprika

Preparation

Dressing: In large bowl, whisk together yogurt, honey, lemon juice, mustard, poppy seeds, salt and paprika until smooth.

Add fennel, celery, grapes and apple; toss to coat. Serve sprinkled with walnuts

Fennel & White Bean Pasta

Ingredients

1 large fennel bulb, trimmed
2 medium zucchini
3 tablespoons extra-virgin olive oil, divided
1/4 teaspoon salt
8 ounces (2 cups) whole-wheat penne or similar short pasta
2 cloves garlic, finely chopped
1 cup cooked cannellini beans, plus 1/2 cup bean-cooking liquid, pasta-cooking liquid or water
2 plum tomatoes, diced
3/4 cup goat cheese
1/4 cup fresh mint leaves
ground pepper to taste

Preparation

Preheat oven to 400 °F. Cut fennel bulb in half lengthwise and then slice lengthwise into 1/2-inch-thick wedges. Quarter zucchini lengthwise. Toss the fennel and zucchini with 1 tablespoon oil and salt. Arrange in a single layer on a large baking sheet. Roast, turning once, until soft and beginning to brown, about 20 minutes. Meanwhile, bring a large pot of water to a boil. Add pasta; cook until just tender, 8 to 10 minutes or according to package directions. Heat the remaining 2 tablespoons oil in a large skillet over medium heat. Add garlic and cook, stirring, for 30 seconds. Remove from the heat. When the vegetables are cool enough to handle, coarsely chop. Add the vegetables, beans and bean-cooking liquid (or other liquid) to the pan with the garlic and place over medium-low heat. Drain the pasta and immediately add it to the pan. Toss thoroughly and add tomatoes; toss until just warm. Remove from the heat and stir in cheese and mint. Season with pepper.

Celery

Calories: 16 per cup

Crunchy, a little salty, packed with fiber and an incredibly high-volume food (meaning you can eat a lot for a few calories), celery is a chef's secret weapon. For almost zero calories it also contains vitamin A, vitamin C, and folate, crucial for a healthy pregnancy.

Celery Salad

Ingredients

8 large celery stalks, stripped of strings
3 tablespoons extra-virgin olive oil
2 tablespoons freshly squeezed lemon juice
4 tablespoons freshly grated Parmesan, plus more for topping
1 1/2 cups cooked cannellini or garbanzo beans, heated
3 tablespoons raisins
1/2 cup sliced almonds, deeply toasted
sea salt
freshly chopped herbs (or herb flowers), or reserved celery leaves

Preparation

Slice the celery stalks quite thinly - 1/8-inch or so. Then, in a small bowl, make a paste with the olive oil, lemon juice, and Parmesan. Set aside. In a large bowl toss the heated beans with the olive-Parmesan mixture. When well combined, add the celery, raisins and most of the almonds. Toss once more. Taste and add a bit of salt if needed. Serve in a bowl or platter topped with herb flowers and/or celery leaves.

Celery Stir Fry

Ingredients

2 Tbsp canola oil
3 small dried chile peppers, broken in half (can sub a 1/8 teaspoon of red chili flakes)
4 cups julienned celery (cut into pieces about 2 inches long)
1-2 Tbsp soy sauce (to taste)
A few drops of dark sesame oil (optional)
Salt and pepper to taste
1 Tbsp sugar

Preparation

Heat the oils and chiles in a wok or frying pan over high heat for 90 seconds, or until the chiles become fragrant and the seeds sizzle.

Add the celery and stir-fry for 3 minutes. Add the soy sauce, sugar and stir-fry one more minute. Drizzle with dark sesame oil if using. Add salt and pepper to taste. Serve hot or at room temperature.

Spicy Shrimp, Celery, and Cashew Stir-fry

Ingredients

2 tablespoon soy sauce
1 tablespoon dark sesame oil
1 -inch piece peeled fresh ginger
3 cloves garlic
1/2 to 1 teaspoon crushed red pepper flakes
2 tablespoons canola oil
4 ribs celery, thinly sliced
3/4 cup roasted salted cashews
3/4 teaspoon salt
1 pound peeled and cleaned medium shrimp

Preparation

Mix the soy sauce and sesame oil in a medium bowl, set aside. Mince the ginger, garlic, and red pepper flakes in a mini chopper.

Heat a large nonstick skillet over high heat until very hot, about 2 minutes. Add 1 tablespoon of the vegetable oil, the celery and cashews. Season with 1/4 teaspoon salt, and stir-fry until the celery turns jade green, about 3 minutes. Transfer the mixture to a plate.

Return the skillet to high heat. Add the remaining 1 tablespoon oil, the shrimp and the remaining 1/2 teaspoon salt, and stir-fry until shrimp turn pink and curl up, about 2 minutes. Add the ginger-garlic mixture and the scallion whites, and stir-fry until fragrant, about 1 minute. Return the celery and cashews to the pan with most of the scallion greens and the reserved soy sauce mixture and stir over the heat for about 1 minute to mix together evenly and blend flavors.

Berries

Calories: 32 per 1/2 cup

Blueberries, raspberries, strawberries—whatever berry you like best—are full of anti-inflammatories, which reduce your risk of heart disease and cancer.

These antioxidant powerhouses are bite-sized immunity boosters, especially when they grow in the wild. In 2007, Cornell University scientists found that wild blueberries contained the most active antioxidants of any fresh fruit, thanks to their high levels of anthocyanins—one of the most potent antioxidants.

Triple Berry Banana Yogurt Smoothie

Ingredients

8 ounces frozen mixed berries
2 small bananas, cut into 2-inch pieces and frozen
6 ounces vanilla yogurt, preferably whole milk
1 cup whole milk
1 to 2 tablespoons honey

Preparation

Add the berries, bananas, yogurt, milk and honey to a blender and puree until smooth. Pour into glasses and serve immediately.

Greek Yogurt Berry Medley Smoothie

Ingredients

1/2 cup sliced strawberries
1/2 cup raspberries
1/2 cup blueberries
1 ripe banana
1 cup Greek yogurt
2 tablespoons old fashioned oats
1-2 tablespoons agave

Preparation

Combine strawberries, raspberries, blueberries, banana, Greek yogurt, oats, agave and 1 cup ice in blender until smooth.

Carrots

Calories: 22 per 1/2 cup

Carrots are very low in saturated fat and cholesterol. It is also a good source of thiamin, niacin, vitamin B6, folate and manganese, and a very good source of dietary fiber, vitamin A, vitamin C, vitamin K, and potassium.

Carrot Cake

Ingredients

3 cups chopped pecans or pecan pieces (1 cup for cake, 2 cups for garnish)
1 and 1/2 cups brown sugar
1/2 cup   granulated sugar
1 cup canola oil
4 large eggs
3/4 cup   smooth unsweetened applesauce
1 teaspoon vanilla extract
2 and 1/2 cups all-purpose flour
2 teaspoons baking powder
1 teaspoon baking soda
1/2 teaspoon salt
1 and 1/2 teaspoons ground cinnamon
1 teaspoon ground ginger
1/4 teaspoon ground nutmeg
1/4 teaspoon ground cloves
2 cups (260g) grated carrots (about 4 large)

Cream Cheese Frosting

16 ounces cream cheese, softened to room temperature
1/2 cup unsalted butter, softened to room temperature
4 cups confectioners sugar
2-3 Tablespoons   heavy cream
1 teaspoon vanilla extract
pinch salt

Preparation

Preheat oven to 300°F degrees. Line a large baking sheet with parchment paper or a silicone baking mat. Spread the chopped pecans on the sheet and toast for 8 minutes. Remove from the oven and allow to cool.

Turn the oven up to 350°F (177°C). Spray two 9-inch cake pans with nonstick spray. Set aside.

In a large bowl, whisk the brown sugar, granulated sugar, oil, eggs, applesauce, and vanilla together until combined and no brown sugar lumps remain. Set aside. In another large bowl, whisk the flour, baking powder, baking soda, salt, cinnamon, ginger, nutmeg, and cloves together until combined. Pour the wet ingredients into the dry ingredients and, using a rubber spatula or wooden spoon, fold the ingredients together until just combined. Then, fold in the carrots and 1 cup of the toasted pecans. The rest of the pecans are used in step 6.

Pour/spoon the batter evenly into the two cake pans. Bake for 30-35 minutes or until a toothpick inserted into the centers comes out clean. Allow the cakes to cool completely in the pans set on a wire rack.

Make the frosting: In a large bowl using a handheld or stand mixer fitted with a whisk or paddle attachment, beat the cream cheese and butter together on medium speed until smooth, about 2 minutes. Add the confectioners sugar and 2 Tablespoons of cream. Beat for 2 minutes. Add the vanilla and 1 more Tablespoon cream if needed to thin out. Beat on high for 2 full minutes. Taste the frosting and add a pinch of salt if it is too sweet.

Assemble and frost: First, using a large serrated knife, layer off the tops of the cakes to create a flat surface. Place 1 cake layer on your cake stand or serving plate. Evenly cover the top with frosting. Top with 2nd layer and spread remaining frosting all over the top and sides. Decorate the sides of the cake with the remaining toasted pecans. Slice and serve.

Honey Glazed Carrots

Ingredients

Salt
1 pound baby carrots
2 tablespoons butter
2 tablespoons honey
1 tablespoon lemon juice
Freshly ground black pepper
1/4 cup chopped flat-leaf parsley

Preparation

In a medium saucepan, bring water to a boil. Add salt and then carrots and cook until tender, 5 to 6 minutes. Drain the carrots and add back to pan with butter, honey and lemon juice. Cook until a glaze coats the carrots, 5 minutes. Season with salt and pepper and garnish with parsley.

Roasted Carrots

Ingredients

12 carrots
3 tablespoons olive oil
1 1⁄4 teaspoons kosher salt
1⁄2 teaspoon fresh ground black pepper
2 tablespoons minced fresh dill or 2 tablespoons parsley

Preparation

Preheat the oven to 400 degrees F.
If the carrots are thick, cut them in half lengthwise; if not, leave whole.
Slice the carrots diagonally in 1 1/2-inch-thick slices.
(The carrots will shrink while cooking so make the slices big.) Toss them in a bowl with the olive oil, salt, and pepper.
Transfer to a sheet pan in 1 layer and roast in the oven for 20 minutes, until browned and tender.
Toss the carrots with minced dill or parsley, season to taste, and serve.

www.ingramcontent.com/pod-product-compliance
Lightning Source LLC
Chambersburg PA
CBHW070204290526
45789CB00002B/903